I0416724

ALASKAPOX
OUTBREAK

From Diagnosis to Public Health Solutions:
Strategies, Remedies, and Insights for
Addressing the Emerging Threat

Sophia Hawthorne

Table of Contents

Introduction

The emergence of novel infectious diseases has always posed a significant threat to public health. Among the myriad of pathogens that have arisen over the centuries, viruses hold a particularly notorious place due to their ability to rapidly spread and cause severe illness. One such virus that has recently garnered attention is the Alaskapox virus, a member of the Orthopoxvirus genus.

Overview of Alaskapox Virus

The Alaskapox virus is a relatively newly discovered virus that belongs to the Orthopoxvirus genus, a group of viruses known to infect and cause disease in humans and animals. The first documented case of

Alaskapox virus occurred in July 2015 when a woman presented with lesions containing an Orthopox virus at a clinic in Fairbanks, Alaska. Subsequent genetic analysis revealed that the virus was a novel Orthopox virus, distinct from other known members of the genus.

Alaskapox virus is characterized by its ability to cause small lesions on the skin, which typically heal within a few weeks. However, in some cases, the lesions may take longer to resolve, as evidenced by the experience of the first known patient who reported that it took six months for the lesion to fully heal. In addition to skin lesions, other reported symptoms include joint or muscle pain and swollen lymph nodes.

The exact mode of transmission of Alaskapox virus to humans remains unclear, although it is hypothesized to be via small animals. Despite the limited number of reported cases, the potential for further spread of the virus underscores the importance of continued research and surveillance efforts.

Historical Background

The discovery of the Alaskapox virus marks a significant milestone in the field of virology, but it also serves as a reminder of the ongoing threat posed by emerging infectious diseases. Throughout history, humanity has faced numerous pandemics and epidemics caused by various pathogens, including viruses, bacteria, and parasites.

One of the most notorious viral diseases in human history is smallpox, caused by the variola virus. Smallpox was responsible for millions of deaths worldwide and left many survivors with severe scarring and lifelong disabilities. Despite its devastating impact, smallpox is also notable for being the first human disease to be eradicated through vaccination efforts led by the World Health Organization (WHO).

The successful eradication of smallpox demonstrates the power of vaccination and coordinated public health interventions in controlling infectious diseases. However, the emergence of new viral threats, such as Alaskapox virus, serves as a sobering reminder that infectious diseases continue to pose a significant challenge to global health security.

In recent years, other members of the Orthopoxvirus genus, such as monkeypox and cowpox, have also attracted attention due to their ability to cause outbreaks in humans.

These viruses highlight the importance of ongoing surveillance and research to better understand their transmission dynamics, clinical manifestations, and potential countermeasures.

In conclusion, the discovery of the Alaskapox virus underscores the need for vigilance and preparedness in the face of emerging infectious diseases. By learning from past experiences and leveraging advances in science and technology, we can better mitigate the impact of future outbreaks and safeguard public health on a global scale.

Chapter 1: Discovery and Epidemiology

The discovery and epidemiology of the Alaskapox virus represent a fascinating journey into understanding the emergence and spread of a novel infectious agent. From its initial identification in Alaska to subsequent cases and spread to other regions, the story of Alaskapox sheds light on the complex dynamics of infectious disease transmission and highlights the importance of surveillance and response efforts in controlling outbreaks.

Initial Discovery in Alaska

The story of Alaskapox begins in July 2015 when a woman visited a clinic in Fairbanks, Alaska, with lesions that contained an

Orthopoxvirus. The woman's symptoms prompted concern among healthcare providers due to the potential for a poxvirus infection, a family of viruses known to cause diseases such as smallpox and cowpox. Subsequent laboratory analysis confirmed the presence of a novel Orthopox virus in the woman's lesions, marking the first documented case of Alaskapox virus.

The discovery of Alaskapox virus raised several questions among researchers and public health officials. How did the virus emerge? What were its transmission dynamics? Was it capable of causing widespread outbreaks? These questions sparked a flurry of scientific investigation aimed at unraveling the mysteries surrounding this newfound pathogen.

Subsequent Cases and Spread

Following the initial discovery, additional cases of Alaskapox virus began to emerge in the Fairbanks area and beyond. In 2020, the Alaska Department of Health and Social Services announced the second known infection of Alaskapox in another Fairbanks woman. Two more cases were identified in the Fairbanks area in the summer of 2021, indicating a potential pattern of localized transmission within the region.

By February 2024, the number of reported cases had risen to seven, with one additional case reported outside of the Fairbanks North Star Borough in the Kenai Peninsula Borough. This marked the first reported case outside of the initial affected area, raising concerns about the potential for further spread of the virus to other regions of Alaska and beyond.

The spread of Alaskapox virus to new areas underscored the need for enhanced surveillance and control measures to prevent further transmission and mitigate the impact of the outbreak. Public health authorities worked tirelessly to identify and isolate cases, trace contacts, and implement targeted interventions to limit the spread of the virus within affected communities.

Reported Cases and Affected Regions

As of February 2024, a total of seven cases of Alaskapox virus had been reported to the Alaska Section of Epidemiology. Six of these cases occurred in the Fairbanks North Star Borough, while one case was reported in the Kenai Peninsula Borough. The geographic distribution of cases highlighted the localized nature of the outbreak, with the majority of cases clustered within specific regions of Alaska.

While the number of reported cases remained relatively low compared to other infectious diseases, the emergence of Alaskapox virus raised concerns about its potential to cause more widespread outbreaks if left unchecked. Public health authorities closely monitored the situation and implemented measures to prevent further transmission, including public education campaigns, enhanced surveillance, and targeted vaccination efforts.

In conclusion, the discovery and epidemiology of the Alaskapox virus underscored the importance of proactive surveillance and response efforts in detecting and controlling emerging infectious diseases. By studying the transmission dynamics and geographic spread of the virus, researchers and public health officials gained valuable insights into the factors driving outbreaks and the strategies needed to contain them.

Chapter 2: Virus Classification and Characteristics.

Taxonomic Classification

The Alaskapox virus belongs to the Orthopoxvirus genus, a diverse group of viruses within the Poxviridae family. Taxonomically, the Orthopoxvirus genus is classified within the Chitovirales order, Pokkesviricetes class, Nucleocytoviricota phylum, Bamfordvirae kingdom, and Varidnaviria realm. This classification places Alaskapox virus alongside other notable members of the Orthopoxvirus genus, including variola virus (smallpox), vaccinia virus, cowpox virus, and monkeypox virus.

Within the Orthopoxvirus genus, Alaskapox virus exhibits distinct genetic and structural features that distinguish it from other members of the genus. Comparative genomic analysis has revealed unique genetic signatures and evolutionary adaptations that shed light on the virus's origins and evolutionary history.

Genetic Makeup and Structure

The genetic makeup and structure of the Alaskapox virus provide valuable insights into its pathogenicity, transmission dynamics, and host interactions. Like other poxviruses, Alaskapox virus is characterized by its large, linear, double-stranded DNA genome, which encodes a diverse array of proteins involved in viral replication, host immune evasion, and virulence.

The genome of Alaskapox virus consists of hundreds of genes organized into functional modules responsible for various aspects of the viral life cycle. These genes encode essential viral proteins, including those involved in viral entry, genome replication, transcription, and assembly. Comparative genomic analysis has revealed both conserved regions shared with other orthopoxviruses and unique genetic elements specific to Alaskapox virus.

Structurally, Alaskapox virus exhibits typical poxvirus morphology, characterized by a complex brick-shaped virion composed of multiple layers of lipid membranes and viral proteins. The virion measures approximately 200-300 nanometers in diameter and contains a central core containing the viral genome, surrounded by an outer membrane layer studded with viral glycoproteins.

The outer membrane of the virion plays a crucial role in viral entry and host-cell recognition, facilitating attachment to host-cell receptors and fusion with cellular membranes during viral entry. The inner core contains the viral genome complexed with viral proteins and enzymes necessary for viral replication and transcription.

In addition to its structural components, Alaskapox virus possesses a diverse array of viral proteins that interact with host-cell factors to modulate host immune responses and facilitate viral replication. These viral proteins play key roles in evading host immune surveillance, suppressing antiviral defenses, and hijacking cellular machinery for viral replication.

Understanding the genetic makeup and structural features of the Alaskapox virus provides a foundation for further research into its pathogenesis, host interactions, and potential interventions. By elucidating the molecular mechanisms underlying virus-host interactions, researchers can develop novel strategies for diagnosing, treating, and preventing Alaskapox virus infection.

Chapter 3: Signs and Symptoms of Alaskapox Virus Infection

Skin Lesions and Their Characteristics

The hallmark feature of Alaskapox virus infection is the presence of small, raised lesions on the skin, which serve as the primary clinical manifestation of the disease. These lesions typically appear as papules or pustules, ranging in size from a few millimeters to several centimeters in diameter. The lesions may be solitary or clustered and can occur on any part of the body, although they are most commonly observed on the face, extremities, and trunk.

The appearance of the lesions may vary depending on the stage of infection. In the early stages, the lesions may appear as red, inflamed papules or vesicles filled with clear fluid. Over time, the lesions may progress to form pustules or crusts, which eventually rupture and scab over. The healing process of the lesions can be prolonged, with some lesions taking several weeks to fully resolve.

Characteristic features of Alaskapox virus lesions include their round or oval shape, well-defined borders, and absence of surrounding inflammation or erythema. Unlike other poxviruses such as smallpox, which often result in deeply indented or pitted scars, Alaskapox virus lesions typically heal without significant scarring.

Duration and Healing Process

The duration of Alaskapox virus lesions can vary depending on individual factors such as the host's immune response, the severity of the infection, and the presence of underlying medical conditions. In general, the lesions typically follow a predictable course of development, maturation, and resolution over the course of several weeks.

In the initial stages of infection, patients may experience mild itching or discomfort at the site of the lesions. As the lesions progress, they may become more painful or tender, particularly if secondary bacterial infection occurs. Despite their appearance, Alaskapox virus lesions are typically self-limiting and resolve spontaneously without medical intervention in the majority of cases.

The healing process of Alaskapox virus lesions typically involves the gradual resolution of inflammation, reduction in lesion size, and eventual formation of a scab or crust. The scab eventually detaches, revealing underlying healthy skin tissue. Complete resolution of the lesions may take several weeks, with some lesions leaving behind faint discoloration or hyperpigmentation that fades over time.

Associated Symptoms such as Joint or Muscle Pain and Swollen Lymph Nodes

In addition to skin lesions, individuals infected with Alaskapox virus may experience various associated symptoms that can impact their overall health and well-being. Common associated symptoms include joint or muscle pain, which may range from mild discomfort to severe aches and stiffness.

Joint or muscle pain typically accompanies the development of skin lesions and may persist throughout the course of the infection. The exact mechanism underlying the development of joint or muscle pain in Alaskapox virus infection is not fully understood but is thought to be related to the inflammatory response triggered by the virus.

Swollen lymph nodes, or lymphadenopathy, may also occur in individuals infected with Alaskapox virus. Lymphadenopathy is characterized by the enlargement and tenderness of lymph nodes, particularly those located near the site of the skin lesions. The swelling of lymph nodes is indicative of the body's immune response to the viral infection and typically resolves once the infection is cleared.

In conclusion, the signs and symptoms of Alaskapox virus infection encompass a spectrum of dermatologic and systemic manifestations, ranging from characteristic skin lesions to associated symptoms such as joint or muscle pain and swollen lymph nodes. By recognizing the clinical features of the disease, healthcare providers can accurately diagnose and manage Alaskapox virus infection, thereby reducing morbidity and improving patient outcomes.

Chapter 4: Unraveling the Transmission of Alaskapox Virus

Hypothesized Modes of Transmission

The precise mode of transmission of the Alaskapox virus to humans remains a subject of ongoing investigation and debate. While definitive evidence is lacking, several hypotheses have been proposed to elucidate the potential routes of transmission. One prevailing hypothesis suggests that Alaskapox virus is transmitted to humans through contact with infected animals or contaminated environments.

Direct contact with infected animals, such as rodents or other small mammals, may facilitate the transmission of the virus to humans through scratches, bites, or mucous membrane exposure. Additionally, indirect contact with contaminated surfaces or fomites, such as animal bedding or food sources, may also pose a risk of transmission if viral particles are present.

Another hypothesis proposes the possibility of airborne transmission, whereby viral particles are expelled into the air through respiratory secretions or aerosolized droplets and subsequently inhaled by susceptible individuals. While airborne transmission is considered less likely than direct or indirect contact transmission, it cannot be ruled out entirely, particularly in settings with close human-animal interactions or crowded environments.

The role of arthropod vectors, such as mosquitoes or ticks, in the transmission of Alaskapox virus remains uncertain. While some poxviruses are known to be transmitted by arthropod vectors, there is currently no evidence to suggest that Alaskapox virus utilizes this mode of transmission. However, further research is needed to explore the potential involvement of arthropod vectors in the epidemiology of the virus.

Animal Reservoirs and Vectors

Identifying potential animal reservoirs and vectors of the Alaskapox virus is essential for understanding the ecological dynamics of viral transmission and implementing targeted control measures. While the natural reservoir(s) of Alaskapox virus remain(s) unknown, several animal species have been implicated as potential hosts based on epidemiological and serological evidence.

Rodents, particularly ground squirrels and voles, have been proposed as potential reservoirs of Alaskapox virus due to their close proximity to human populations and their known susceptibility to other orthopoxviruses. Serological studies have detected antibodies to orthopoxviruses in rodent populations in Alaska, suggesting past exposure to related viruses.

Other small mammals, such as shrews and bats, have also been considered as potential reservoirs or amplifying hosts for Alaskapox virus. These animals may play a role in maintaining the virus in the environment and facilitating transmission to humans through direct or indirect contact.

Arthropod vectors, including mosquitoes and ticks, have been investigated as potential vehicles for the transmission of Alaskapox virus. While there is limited evidence to support the involvement of arthropod vectors in the transmission of the virus, their role in the ecology of Alaskapox virus warrants further investigation.

Potential Routes of Human Infection

Human infection with Alaskapox virus may occur through various routes, including direct contact with infected animals or contaminated environments, respiratory droplets, or aerosolized particles. Individuals who handle infected animals or come into close contact with their habitats may be at increased risk of infection, particularly if proper precautions are not taken to prevent exposure.

In addition to direct contact transmission, Alaskapox virus may also be transmitted through respiratory secretions or aerosolized droplets expelled by infected individuals. Close proximity to an infected person, particularly in crowded or confined settings, may increase the risk of respiratory transmission.

Furthermore, fomite transmission, whereby viral particles are deposited on surfaces or objects and subsequently transferred to susceptible individuals through hand-to-mouth contact, may also contribute to the spread of Alaskapox virus. Proper hand hygiene and environmental disinfection are essential for reducing the risk of fomite transmission in settings where viral particles may be present.

In conclusion, the transmission dynamics of the Alaskapox virus are complex and multifaceted, involving potential routes of transmission, animal reservoirs, and vectors. Understanding the mechanisms of viral spread is critical for implementing effective control measures and mitigating the impact of the outbreak on human health and well-being. Further research is needed to elucidate the dynamics of Alaskapox virus transmission and inform public health interventions aimed at preventing future outbreaks.

Chapter 5: Diagnosis and Laboratory Testing for Alaskapox Virus

Methods for Identifying Alaskapox Virus

Several laboratory-based methods are available for the identification of Alaskapox virus, each offering unique advantages and limitations in terms of sensitivity, specificity, and turnaround time. These methods include:

1. **Polymerase Chain Reaction (PCR)**: PCR-based assays are commonly used for the molecular detection of viral nucleic acids in clinical specimens. Targeted PCR assays designed to amplify specific regions of the Alaskapox virus genome can provide rapid and sensitive detection of the virus in clinical samples, such as lesion swabs or tissue biopsies.

Real-time PCR assays offer the additional advantage of quantifying viral load, which may be useful for monitoring disease progression and response to treatment.

2. **Virus Isolation**: Virus isolation involves the propagation of the virus in cell culture followed by the detection of viral cytopathic effects or the presence of viral antigens using immunofluorescence or other staining techniques. While virus isolation is considered the gold standard for confirming viral infection, it requires specialized laboratory facilities and may take several days to weeks to yield results.

3. **Serological Assays**: Serological assays detect the presence of antibodies against Alaskapox virus in patient serum or plasma samples. Enzyme-linked immunosorbent assays (ELISAs) and neutralization assays are

commonly used serological techniques for detecting specific antibodies against viral antigens. Serological assays are useful for confirming past exposure to the virus and assessing immune status but may be less sensitive during the acute phase of infection.

4. Next-Generation Sequencing (NGS): NGS technologies enable the high-throughput sequencing of viral genomes directly from clinical specimens, allowing for comprehensive genomic characterization of the virus. NGS can provide valuable insights into the genetic diversity, evolution, and transmission dynamics of Alaskapox virus, facilitating epidemiological investigations and outbreak surveillance.

5. Immunohistochemistry (IHC): IHC staining of tissue sections using specific antibodies against viral antigens can aid in the histopathological diagnosis of Alaskapox virus infection. IHC allows for the visualization of viral antigens within infected tissues, providing valuable diagnostic information for pathologists and clinicians.

Differential Diagnosis with Other Poxviruses

Distinguishing Alaskapox virus infection from other poxvirus infections, such as variola virus (smallpox), monkeypox virus, and cowpox virus, can be challenging due to the overlapping clinical and histopathological features of these diseases. Several factors should be considered when making a differential diagnosis, including:

1. **Clinical Presentation**: While Alaskapox virus infection typically presents with small,

raised skin lesions, the clinical presentation may vary depending on the severity of the disease and the individual's immune status. Variola virus infection, in contrast, often manifests as a generalized rash with characteristic stages of lesion development, including papules, vesicles, pustules, and scabs.

2. **Epidemiological Context**: The epidemiological context of the case, including the geographic location, travel history, and known exposure to animals or other individuals with similar symptoms, can provide valuable clues for differential diagnosis. For example, cases of monkeypox virus infection are often associated with exposure to infected animals or travelers returning from endemic regions.

3. **Laboratory Testing**: Laboratory testing, including PCR, virus isolation, serological

assays, and histopathological examination, can help differentiate Alaskapox virus infection from other poxvirus infections. Molecular techniques, such as PCR and NGS, can provide specific identification of the virus based on its genetic sequence, while serological assays can detect specific antibodies against viral antigens.

4.   **Histopathological   Findings**: Histopathological examination of skin biopsy specimens can reveal characteristic features of poxvirus infection, including epidermal hyperplasia, ballooning degeneration of keratinocytes, intracytoplasmic inclusion bodies, and perivascular lymphocytic infiltrates. However, these findings may be nonspecific and require confirmation through additional laboratory testing.

In conclusion, accurate diagnosis of Alaskapox virus infection requires a multifaceted approach, combining clinical evaluation, laboratory testing, and epidemiological investigation. By employing a comprehensive diagnostic strategy, healthcare providers can effectively identify and manage cases of Alaskapox virus infection, thereby reducing morbidity and mortality associated with the disease.

Chapter 6: Treatment and Management of Alaskapox Virus Infection

Current Treatment Options

As of now, there are no specific antiviral medications approved for the treatment of Alaskapox virus infection. However, supportive care measures and symptomatic management play a crucial role in alleviating symptoms and promoting recovery in affected individuals. These supportive measures may include:

1.   Pain   Management: Nonsteroidal anti-inflammatory   drugs   (NSAIDs)   or acetaminophen may be used to alleviate pain and reduce fever associated with Alaskapox virus infection. These medications can help

improve patient comfort and facilitate restful sleep during the acute phase of the illness.

2. Fluid and Electrolyte Replacement: Maintaining adequate hydration and electrolyte balance is essential for patients with Alaskapox virus infection, particularly those with severe dehydration or electrolyte imbalances due to fever, vomiting, or diarrhea. Oral rehydration solutions or intravenous fluids may be administered as needed to prevent dehydration and support recovery.

3. Wound Care: Proper wound care is essential for preventing secondary bacterial infections and promoting the healing of skin lesions associated with Alaskapox virus infection. Antiseptic solutions or topical antibiotics may be applied to the affected areas to prevent

bacterial colonization and facilitate wound healing.

4. Isolation and Infection Control: Implementing strict isolation precautions and infection control measures is essential for preventing the spread of Alaskapox virus infection to other individuals. Infected individuals should be isolated from non-infected individuals, and healthcare providers should adhere to standard precautions when caring for patients with suspected or confirmed Alaskapox virus infection.

Supportive Care and Symptom Management

In addition to the aforementioned treatment options, supportive care and symptom management play a crucial role in the overall management of Alaskapox virus infection. Supportive care measures aim to address the specific needs of individual patients and improve their overall comfort and well-being. These measures may include:

1. Nutritional Support: Providing adequate nutrition is essential for supporting the immune system and promoting recovery in patients with Alaskapox virus infection. Nutrient-rich foods, oral nutritional supplements, or enteral feeding may be recommended for patients who are unable to meet their nutritional needs through oral intake alone.

2. Psychosocial Support: Coping with the physical and emotional challenges of Alaskapox virus infection can be difficult for patients and

their families. Psychosocial support services, such as counseling, support groups, or peer-to-peer support networks, can provide valuable emotional support and guidance to individuals affected by the disease.

3. Respiratory Support: In severe cases of Alaskapox virus infection associated with respiratory compromise, supplemental oxygen therapy or mechanical ventilation may be required to support respiratory function and ensure adequate oxygenation of tissues.

4. Rehabilitation Services: Patients recovering from Alaskapox virus infection may benefit from rehabilitation services, such as physical therapy, occupational therapy, or speech therapy, to regain strength, mobility, and functional independence.

Potential Future Developments in Treatment

While current treatment options for Alaskapox virus infection are limited to supportive care and symptomatic management, ongoing research efforts hold promise for the development of novel therapeutic interventions. Potential future developments in the treatment of Alaskapox virus infection may include:

1. Antiviral Therapies: The identification of specific antiviral agents targeting key viral proteins or pathways involved in viral replication and pathogenesis could lead to the development of effective antiviral therapies for Alaskapox virus infection. Screening of existing antiviral drugs or the development of new antiviral compounds through rational drug design approaches may offer promising avenues for therapeutic intervention.

2. Immunomodulatory Therapies: Modulation of the host immune response to Alaskapox virus infection through the administration of immunomodulatory agents, such as interferons, cytokines, or monoclonal antibodies, may help enhance antiviral immunity and reduce disease severity. Immunomodulatory therapies could potentially be used in combination with antiviral drugs to achieve synergistic effects and improve treatment outcomes.

3. Vaccine Development: Development of a safe and effective vaccine against Alaskapox virus could provide long-term protection against infection and help prevent future outbreaks of the disease. Vaccine candidates could be based on live attenuated viruses, viral subunit proteins, or viral vectors expressing Alaskapox virus antigens, with the goal of eliciting robust

and durable immune responses in vaccinated individuals.

In conclusion, while current treatment options for Alaskapox virus infection are limited to supportive care and symptomatic management, ongoing research efforts offer hope for the development of novel therapeutic interventions in the future. By advancing our understanding of the virus's pathogenesis and host immune response, researchers can identify new targets for therapeutic intervention and accelerate the development of effective treatments for this emerging infectious disease.

Chapter 7: Prevention and Control of Alaskapox Virus Infection

Vaccination Strategies

Developing a safe and effective vaccine against Alaskapox virus is a key priority in the prevention and control of the disease. Vaccination strategies aim to induce protective immunity against the virus, thereby reducing the risk of infection and limiting the spread of the disease within susceptible populations. Several potential vaccine candidates and vaccination approaches may be considered, including:

1. Live Attenuated Vaccines: Live attenuated vaccines containing weakened or modified strains of Alaskapox virus could stimulate a

robust immune response while minimizing the risk of disease. Live attenuated vaccines mimic natural infection and provide long-lasting immunity against the virus. However, safety concerns regarding potential reversion to virulence and adverse effects must be carefully evaluated in preclinical and clinical studies.

2. Subunit Vaccines: Subunit vaccines consist of purified viral proteins or antigenic components derived from Alaskapox virus. These vaccines offer the advantage of enhanced safety and specificity, as they do not contain live virus particles. Subunit vaccines can be produced using recombinant DNA technology or protein expression systems and may be formulated with adjuvants to enhance immunogenicity.

3. Viral Vector Vaccines: Viral vector vaccines utilize non-pathogenic viral vectors, such as

adenoviruses or poxviruses, to deliver genes encoding Alaskapox virus antigens into host cells. Viral vector vaccines induce strong cellular and humoral immune responses against the target virus and have the potential for rapid development and scalability. However, concerns regarding pre-existing immunity to the viral vector and vector-related adverse effects must be addressed.

4. DNA Vaccines: DNA vaccines consist of plasmid DNA encoding viral antigens, which are administered directly into host cells to stimulate an immune response. DNA vaccines offer the advantages of simplicity, stability, and ease of production and distribution. DNA vaccines can be engineered to express specific Alaskapox virus antigens and may be administered via intramuscular or intradermal injection.

Public Health Measures for Containment

In addition to vaccination strategies, public health measures play a critical role in containing the spread of Alaskapox virus infection and mitigating the impact of the outbreak. Public health interventions aim to reduce transmission within affected communities, identify and isolate cases, and implement targeted control measures to limit the spread of the virus. Key public health measures for containment may include:

1. Surveillance and Early Detection: Implementing robust surveillance systems to monitor for cases of Alaskapox virus infection and identify clusters of illness within communities. Early detection of cases allows for

prompt intervention and implementation of control measures to prevent further spread of the virus.

2. Case Isolation and Contact Tracing: Isolating confirmed cases of Alaskapox virus infection and tracing contacts of infected individuals to identify potential sources of transmission and secondary cases. Quarantine measures may be implemented for individuals exposed to the virus to prevent further spread within the community.

3. Personal Protective Measures: Promoting personal protective measures, such as hand hygiene, respiratory etiquette, and wearing of face masks, to reduce the risk of transmission of Alaskapox virus and other respiratory pathogens. Educating the public about the

importance of these measures can help prevent the spread of the virus in community settings.

4. Environmental Disinfection: Implementing rigorous environmental cleaning and disinfection protocols in healthcare facilities, public spaces, and high-risk settings to reduce the environmental reservoir of the virus and prevent transmission through contaminated surfaces or fomites.

Recommendations for At-Risk Populations

Certain populations may be at increased risk of Alaskapox virus infection due to factors such as occupational exposure, travel to endemic areas, or underlying medical conditions. Recommendations for at-risk populations may include:

1. Occupational Health and Safety Measures: Implementing occupational health and safety measures to protect healthcare workers, laboratory personnel, and individuals working in close contact with animals or animal products from potential exposure to Alaskapox virus. These measures may include the use of personal protective equipment, vaccination, and adherence to infection control protocols.

2. Travel Advisories and Precautions: Providing travel advisories and recommendations for individuals traveling to regions where Alaskapox virus infection is endemic or where outbreaks have occurred. Travelers should be advised to avoid contact with sick or dead animals, practice good hygiene, and seek medical attention if they develop symptoms suggestive of Alaskapox virus infection.

3. Vaccination Campaigns: Targeted vaccination campaigns may be implemented to vaccinate at-risk populations, such as healthcare workers, first responders, and individuals living or working in high-risk areas, against Alaskapox virus infection. Vaccination efforts should be coordinated with public health authorities and tailored to the specific needs and risk factors of the target population.

4. Public Health Education and Awareness: Educating the public about the signs and symptoms of Alaskapox virus infection, transmission routes, and preventive measures through public health campaigns

Chapter 8: Research and Future Directions in Alaskapox Virus

Ongoing Research Efforts

Research on Alaskapox virus spans multiple disciplines, including virology, epidemiology, immunology, and public health, with ongoing efforts aimed at elucidating the fundamental aspects of the virus and developing strategies for its prevention and control. Current research initiatives include:

1. Epidemiological Studies: Epidemiological studies are underway to characterize the geographic distribution, prevalence, and risk factors associated with Alaskapox virus infection. These studies aim to identify patterns of transmission, high-risk populations, and

environmental factors contributing to the spread of the virus.

2. Virological Investigations: Virological investigations focus on characterizing the genetic diversity, molecular epidemiology, and host-virus interactions of Alaskapox virus. Genomic sequencing studies provide insights into the evolutionary history, virulence determinants, and antigenic variability of the virus, informing vaccine development and diagnostic strategies.

3. Pathogenesis Studies: Pathogenesis studies aim to elucidate the mechanisms underlying Alaskapox virus infection, host immune response, and disease progression. Animal models, such as mice or non-human primates, may be used to study the pathogenesis of the

virus and evaluate candidate vaccines and therapeutics.

4. Diagnostic Development: Development of sensitive and specific diagnostic assays for the detection of Alaskapox virus infection is a priority for research efforts. Novel molecular, serological, and imaging techniques may be explored to improve diagnostic accuracy and facilitate early detection of cases.

5. Vaccine Development: Vaccine development efforts focus on the design and evaluation of candidate vaccines against Alaskapox virus. Preclinical studies assess the safety, immunogenicity, and efficacy of vaccine candidates in animal models, paving the way for clinical trials in humans.

Areas for Further Investigation

Despite significant progress, several key areas require further investigation to advance our understanding of Alaskapox virus and inform public health interventions. Areas for further investigation include:

1. Transmission Dynamics: Further research is needed to elucidate the modes of transmission, reservoir hosts, and environmental factors contributing to the spread of Alaskapox virus. Understanding the dynamics of viral transmission is critical for implementing targeted control measures and preventing future outbreaks.

2. Immune Response: Studies investigating the immune response to Alaskapox virus infection are essential for identifying correlates of protection, understanding immune evasion

mechanisms, and developing effective vaccines and therapeutics. Characterizing the host immune response may also inform treatment strategies and prognostic markers.

3. Antiviral Therapies: Development of specific antiviral therapies targeting Alaskapox virus is a priority for research efforts. Screening of existing antiviral compounds, repurposing of drugs with known antiviral activity, and development of novel therapeutics hold promise for the treatment of Alaskapox virus infection.

4. Surveillance and Outbreak Response: Enhanced surveillance systems and rapid outbreak response capabilities are essential for early detection and containment of Alaskapox virus outbreaks. Research on innovative surveillance technologies, data analytics, and

predictive modeling can improve our ability to detect and respond to emerging threats.

Potential Challenges and Opportunities in Alaskapox Research

While research on Alaskapox virus offers significant opportunities for scientific discovery and public health impact, several challenges must be addressed to advance the field effectively. Potential challenges and opportunities in Alaskapox research include:

1. Limited Resources: Limited funding, infrastructure, and expertise may hinder research efforts on Alaskapox virus, particularly in resource-limited settings. Collaborative partnerships, interdisciplinary research teams, and international cooperation can leverage

resources and expertise to address research priorities effectively.

2. Ethical Considerations: Research involving infectious agents such as Alaskapox virus raises ethical considerations related to biosafety, biosecurity, and informed consent. Ethical guidelines and oversight mechanisms are essential to ensure that research is conducted responsibly, transparently, and ethically.

3. Emerging Variants: Ongoing surveillance for emerging variants of Alaskapox virus is critical for monitoring changes in virulence, transmissibility, and antigenicity that may impact vaccine efficacy and diagnostic accuracy. Genomic surveillance networks and global collaborations can facilitate real-time monitoring of viral diversity and inform public health interventions.

4. Global Health Equity: Ensuring equitable access to research resources, diagnostic tools, and vaccines for Alaskapox virus is essential for addressing global health disparities and promoting health equity. Research initiatives should prioritize the needs of underserved populations and vulnerable communities to mitigate the impact of the disease on disadvantaged groups.

In conclusion, research on Alaskapox virus is a dynamic and multidisciplinary field that holds great promise for advancing our understanding of this emerging infectious disease and developing effective strategies for its prevention and control. By addressing key research priorities, overcoming challenges, and fostering collaboration and innovation, researchers can contribute to the global effort to combat Alaskapox virus and protect public health.

Conclusion: Advancing Understanding and Addressing Challenges in Alaskapox Virus Research

Summary of Key Findings

Alaskapox virus, a novel orthopoxvirus species first documented in Alaska in 2015, has emerged as a cause of human illness, with several reported cases in the Fairbanks North Star Borough and Kenai Peninsula Borough. The virus is characterized by small skin lesions, joint or muscle pain, and swollen lymph nodes, with transmission hypothesized to occur through contact with infected animals or contaminated environments. While there are no specific antiviral therapies for Alaskapox virus infection, supportive care measures and symptomatic management play a crucial role in alleviating symptoms and promoting recovery. Vaccination strategies, public health measures for containment, and recommendations for at-risk populations are essential for preventing the spread of the virus and minimizing its impact on public health.

Implications for Public Health and Disease Prevention

The findings presented in this exploration have several implications for public health and disease prevention:

1. Surveillance and Early Detection: Robust surveillance systems are essential for early detection of Alaskapox virus cases and prompt intervention to prevent further spread of the virus. Enhanced surveillance efforts, including

active case finding, syndromic surveillance, and environmental monitoring, can improve our ability to detect and respond to outbreaks in real time.

2. Vaccination and Immunization: Developing safe and effective vaccines against Alaskapox virus is a priority for disease prevention. Vaccination campaigns targeting at-risk populations, healthcare workers, and individuals living or working in high-risk areas can help prevent the spread of the virus and protect vulnerable individuals from infection.

3. Infection Control Measures: Implementing infection control measures, such as isolation of confirmed cases, contact tracing, personal protective equipment, and environmental disinfection, is essential for preventing transmission of Alaskapox virus in healthcare

settings and community settings. Adherence to standard precautions and infection control protocols can minimize the risk of secondary transmission and protect healthcare workers and the public.

4. Public Health Education and Awareness: Educating the public about the signs and symptoms of Alaskapox virus infection, transmission routes, preventive measures, and vaccination recommendations is crucial for raising awareness and promoting behavior change. Public health campaigns, community outreach initiatives, and educational materials can empower individuals to take proactive steps to protect themselves and their communities from infection.

In conclusion, Alaskapox virus represents a significant public health threat that requires coordinated efforts from researchers, healthcare providers, public health authorities, policymakers, and communities to mitigate its impact and prevent further spread. By advancing our understanding of the virus, implementing evidence-based interventions, and fostering collaboration and innovation, we can effectively combat Alaskapox virus and protect the health and well-being of individuals and populations worldwide.